NICOLE SCHEAFBAUER, RD LD

Low Carb Crash Course

5 Easy Ways To Make Changes That Will Stick

This book was professionally typeset on Reedsy.
Find out more at reedsy.com

Contents

Introduction

Hello and welcome to my low carb crash course on how to make low carb eating a breeze for you! Let me first introduce myself…My name is Nicole and I started my career back in 1995 as a registered dietitian and worked as a clinical dietitian in a hospital for ten years where I learned the ropes. I have worked in an OBGYN clinic for four years specializing in helping patients with PCOS, gestational diabetes and general weight loss. My most rewarding outcomes have been helping my PCOS patients lose weight and have babies, helping my patients reverse diabetes, get off medications and just feel better!

Currently I am working in a bariatric clinic helping patients prepare for their pre and post-surgical diets! I love to hear all of their non-scale victories and how excited they are to be able to do the things they never could before.

In a nutshell, all of my rewarding patient outcomes have all been related to limiting carbohydrate intake. This is the reason why I want to write this book for you! As a society we are eating WAY TOO MANY CARBS! So let's get started!

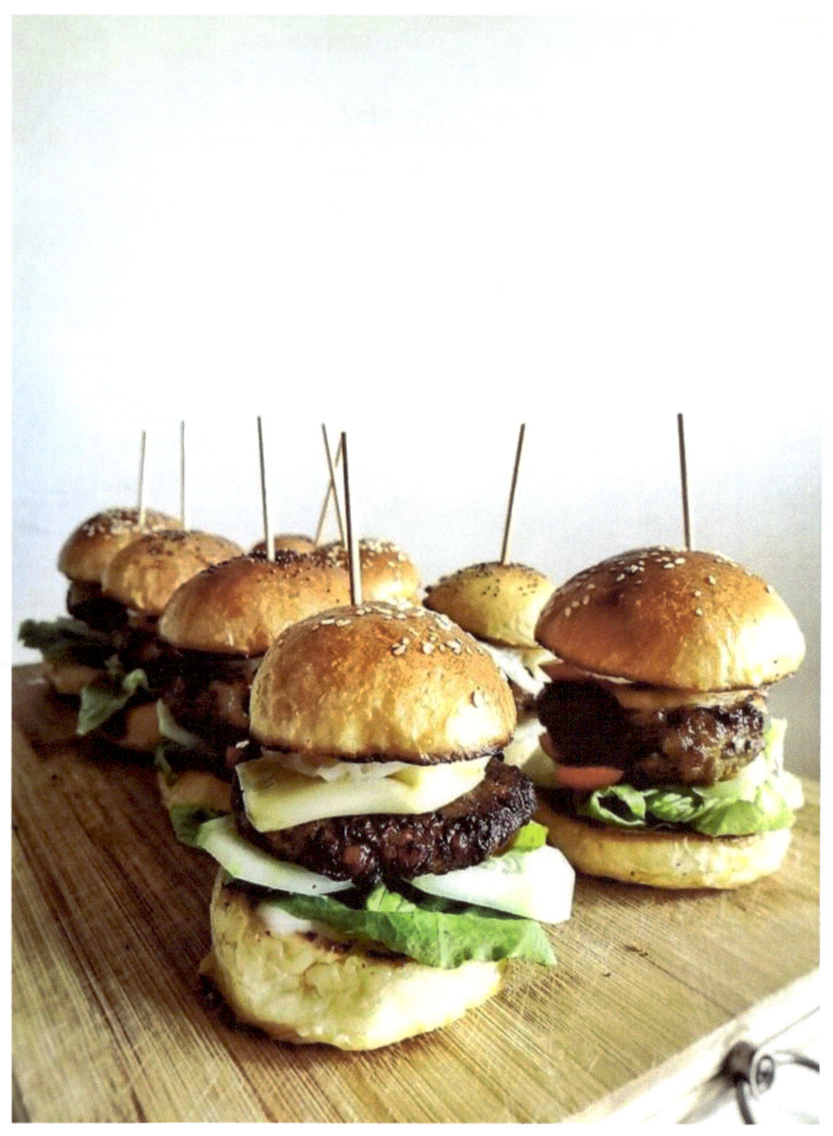

1

How Many Carbs Do You Really Need?

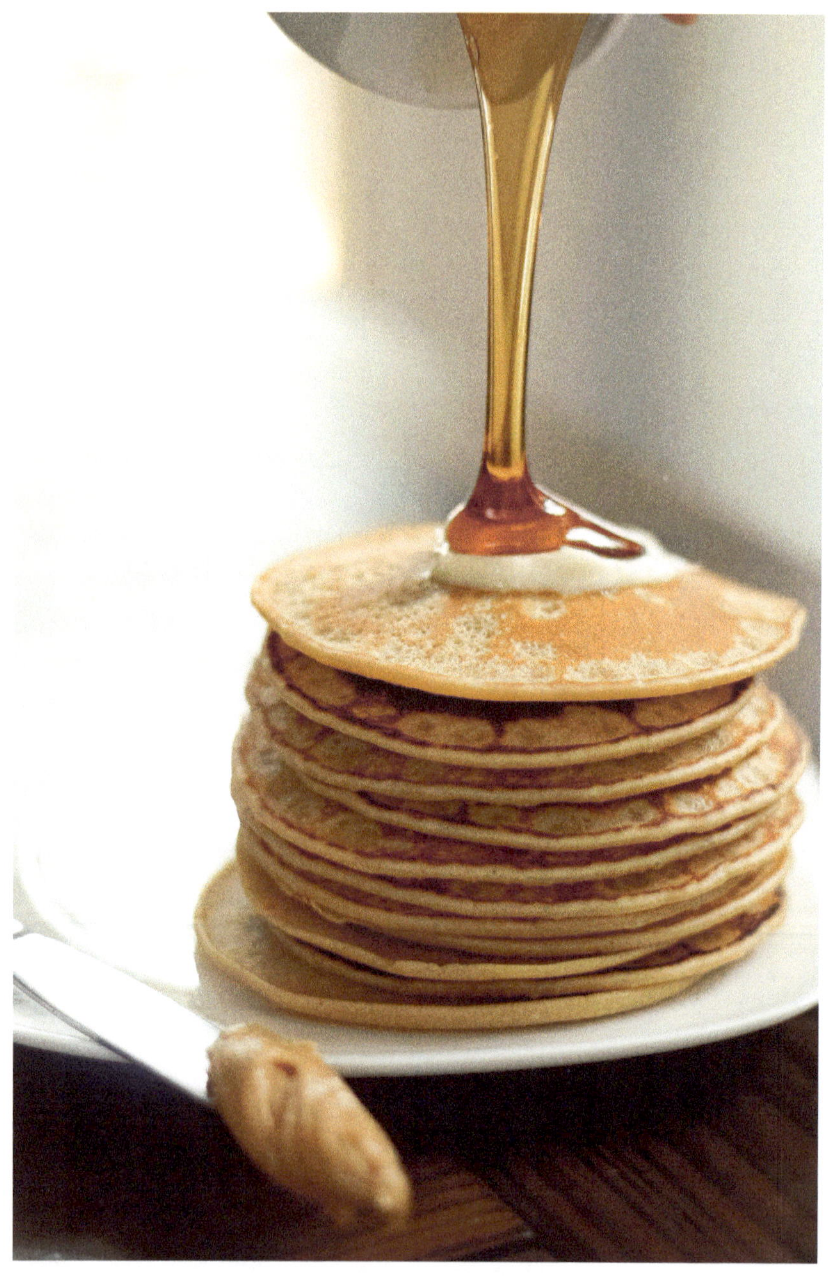

Your body only needs one teaspoon of sugar, also known as glucose, in your daily blood. What happens to the rest of the carbohydrates you eat? They are converted into glucose in your body, some is stored in your muscles and equivalent to 100 grams of carbs are stored in your liver.

So what happens to the excess glucose floating around in your blood? It all converts to storage, thanks to the help of a hormone called insulin. Your pancreas secretes insulin every time you eat carbohydrates. When insulin is overwhelmed with too much glucose, it parks it in storage, otherwise known as your fat. In general, women should be eating less than 100, and men less than 200, total grams of carbohydrates in a day.

What Else Do Carbs Do in Your Body?

If you want to help avoid water retention, you have to limit carbs! This is why you can get on the scale after a day of heavy carb intake and it looks like you've gained 3-5 pounds. You did not gain that many pounds from one meal. Actually, for every gram of carbohydrate you eat, your body retains 3 to 4 grams of water to help store carbs as glycogen for energy. When you cut back on your carbs, or follow a keto diet, your body will naturally diurese and get rid of fluid. This will contribute to some of your initial weight loss. You will feel so much better!

Carbs may also cause bloating and gas. Some of you may have a slight intolerance to carbohydrates and some of you may not. Carbs can be poorly digested and end up being fermented by gut microbes. This causes gas to build up in the large intestine, contributing to 'bloated' feelings. For me personally, if I eat a lot of non fiber-containing carbohydrates, I will feel miserable with bloating and gas. I feel so much better when I follow a low carb intake.

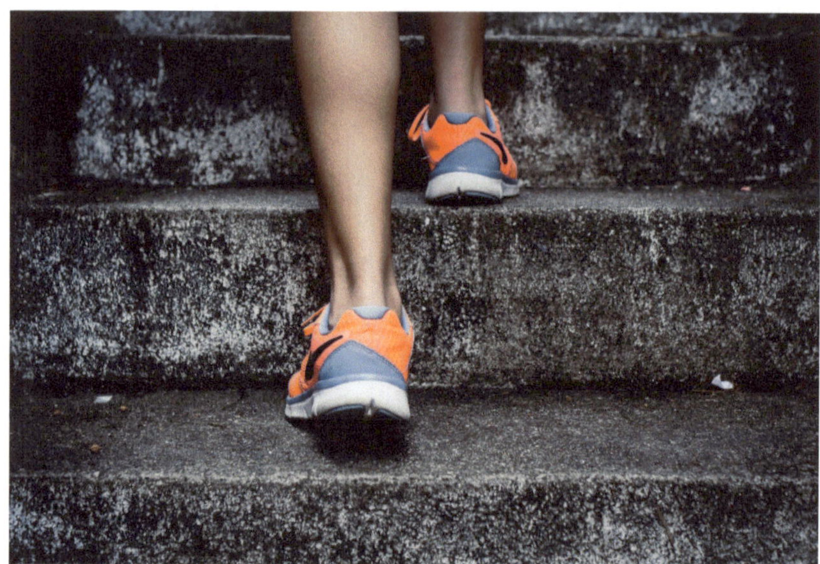

Chasing Your Excess Carb Intake With Cardio Exercise

Truth be told! You can't exercise away your excess carbohydrate intake! What you eat contributes to 90% of your current weight. Exercise and your genetics contribute to the remaining 10% of your weight. This is why following a low carbohydrate intake is so very important!

When I was in college studying to be a dietitian, I was taught that "low fat"eating was all that mattered to be healthy and to avoid a heart attack. I would work out twice a day at the gym, go on long runs and do aerobic classes. Why was I getting fat? I will tell you why! It was because I was eating low fat, trying to be healthy, and instead ate tons of high carb foods! I had to do my own research to figure out it was the carbohydrates causing myself to gain weight, not the fats. Cardio exercise alone will not cause weight loss. If you think you can eat a lot of carbohydrates because you exercise, you are not going to lose weight. You cannot exercise away a high carb intake. Cardio exercise is good for your heart and mental health. I do recommend strength training to maintain your lean muscle mass. This will increase your overall metabolic health. Another eye opener was when I was 29 years old I ran a marathon and looked around me and wondered why so many people were overweight running a marathon? Ah, now it all makes sense!

2

What Foods Are Carbohydrates?

With all the low carb and keto hype, I still have patients who are not aware of which foods are carbohydrate foods. Therefore, I am going to provide you with lists of carbohydrate-containing foods for your reference before you go any further into the book.

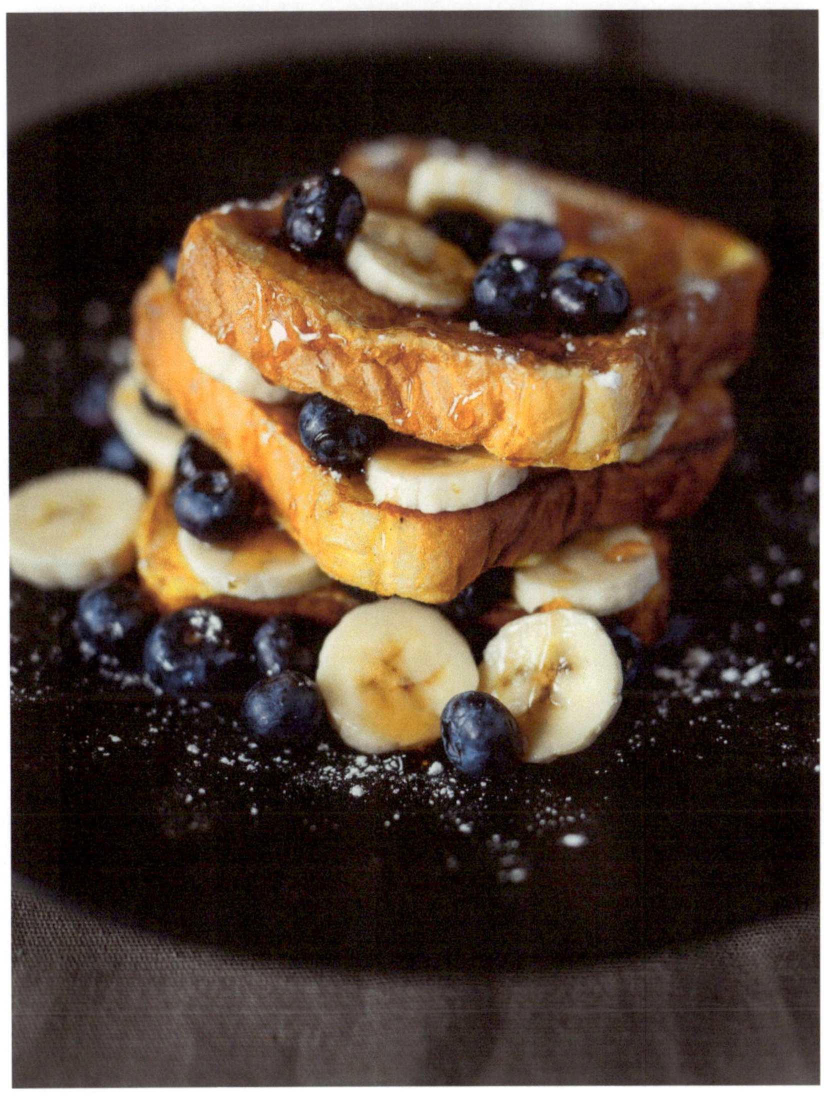

Let's Start with Simple Carbohydrates. These convert into sugar faster in your blood and are added to **sweets** and **desserts** that provide no nutrients:

- Table Sugar
- Cane Sugar
- Invert Sugar
- Molasses
- Confectioner's Sugar
- High Fructose Corn Syrup
- Dextrose
- Brown Sugar
- Sugar-in-the Raw
- Maple Syrup
- Honey
- Malt
- Corn Sweeteners
- Sucrose, Maltose

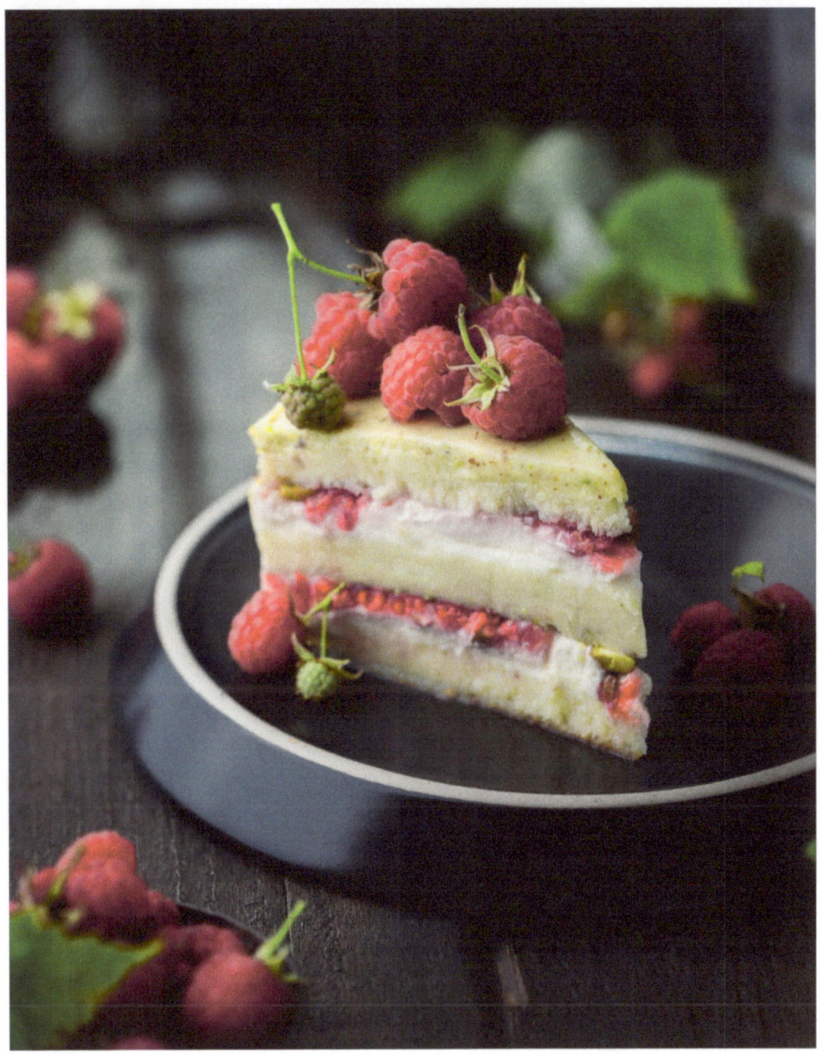

YES! Fruits and milk are natural simple carbohydrates that contain some nutrients but are still converted into glucose in your blood.

Each serving contains approximately 15 grams of carbohydrates:

1 Apple, small

1/2 cup Applesauce, unsweetened

8 halves, 4 whole Apricots

1/2 large Banana

3/4 cup Blackberries

1 cup Cantaloupe

12 Cherries

3 Dates

2 Tbsp Dried fruits

1/2 cup Fruit cocktail

1/2 Grapefruit

17 Grapes, small

1 cup Honeydew melon

1 Kiwi

3/4 cup Mandarin oranges

1/2 cup Mango, small

1 Nectarine, small

1 Orange, small

1 Peach, small

1 Pear, small

1/2 cup Pineapple

2 Plums, small

1/2 cup Raspberries

1 1/3 cup whole Strawberries

2 Tangerines, small

1 1/4 cup Watermelon

8 oz Milk

6 oz yogurt

Put Your Brake on Processed Carbohydrates! Not the best carbs to choose either. You can read the label for portion size and total grams of carbohydrates:

- Bagel
- Biscuit
- Bread
- Chapati
- Cornbread
- English Muffin
- Hot Dog Bun
- Hamburger Bun
- Pancake
- Pita
- Cereals
- Hot Cereals
- Barley
- Bulgar
- Roll
- Stuffing
- Taco Shell
- Tortilla
- Waffle
- Crackers
- Graham Crackers
- Melba Toast
- Oyster Crackers
- Popcorn
- Pretzels
- Chips
- Granola

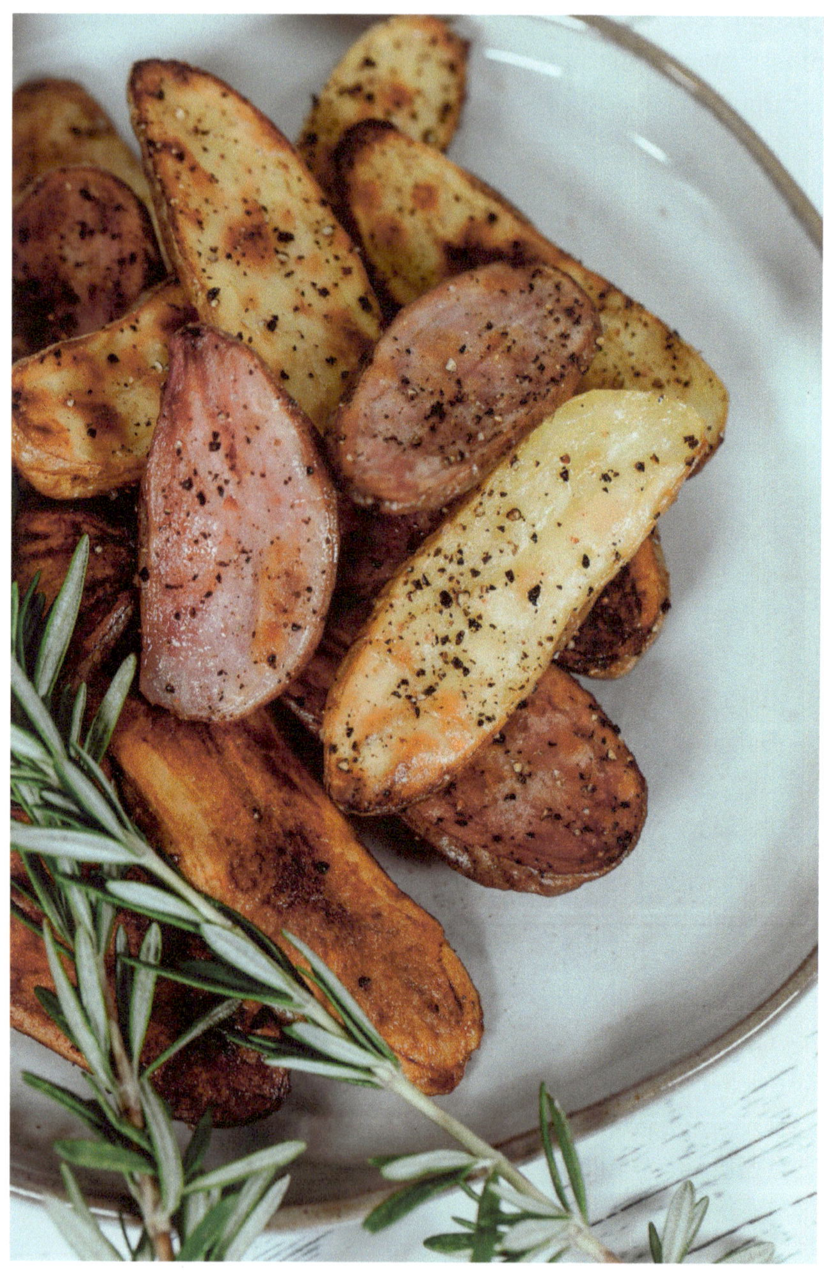

Starchy Vegetables are Carbohydrates! Each serving contains approximately 15 grams of carbs:

- Corn ½ cup
- Corn on the Cob ½ ear
- Hominy ½ cup
- Mixed Vegetables 1 cup
- Parsnips ½ cup
- Green Peas ½ cup
- Ripe Plantain ½ cup
- Baked Potato, medium ½ each
- Boiled Potato ½ cup
- Mashed Potato ½ cup
- French Fries 1 cup
- Pumpkin, canned unsweetened 1 cup
- Red Pasta Sauce 1 cup
- Winter, Acorn, Butternut Squash ½ cup
- Sweet Potato, medium ½ each

Low Carb Intake & Fiber

You can still get sufficient fiber intake while eating a low carb intake. The combination carb foods list below contains good sources of fiber. Non-starchy vegetables such as broccoli, cauliflower, brussel sprouts, asparagus, zucchini and carrots, are also excellent sources of dietary fiber.

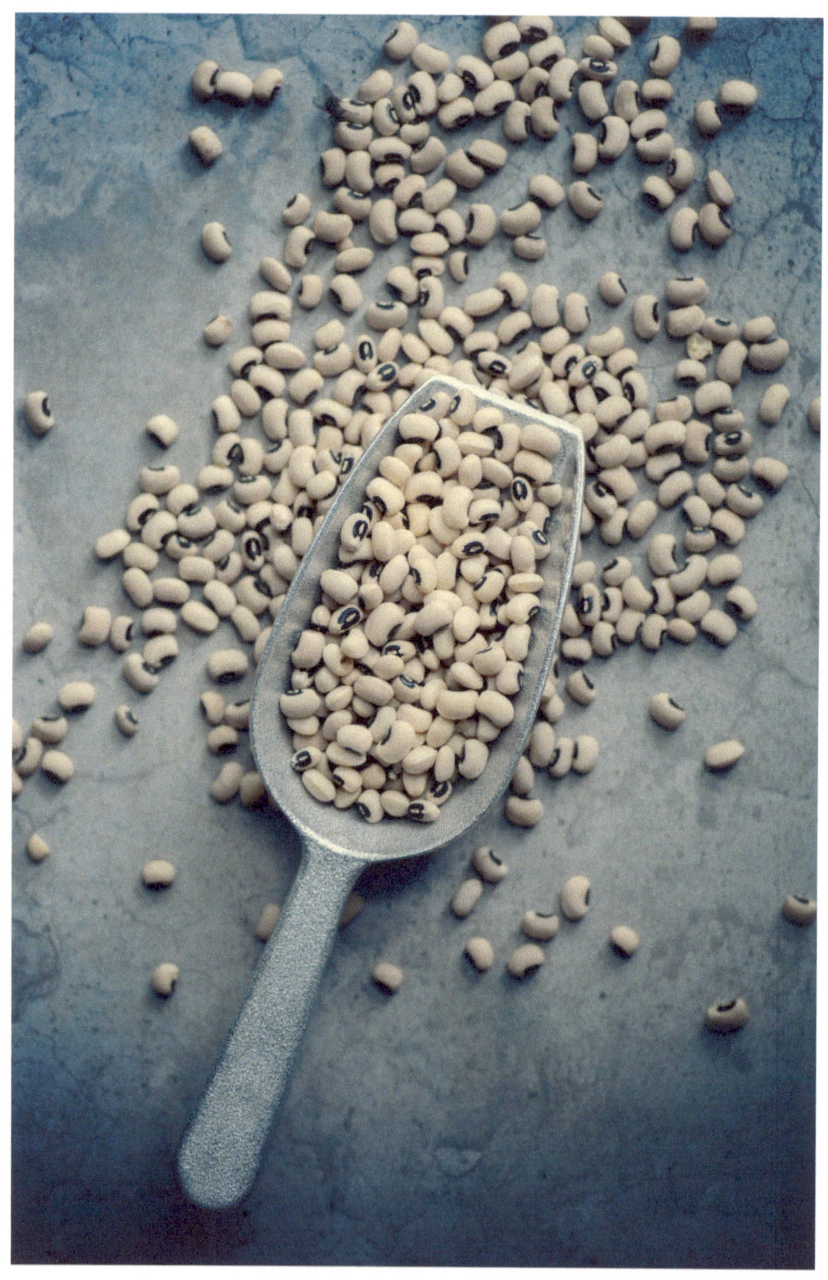

Combination Carb Foods
These foods contain protein, and are good sources of fiber!

- Baked Beans
- Cooked black, garbanzo, kidney, lima, navy, pinto, white beans
- Cooked brown, green, yellow lentils
- Cooked black-eyed split peas
- Refried Beans
- Hummus
- Edamame
- Nuts, Seeds
- Meatless Burger

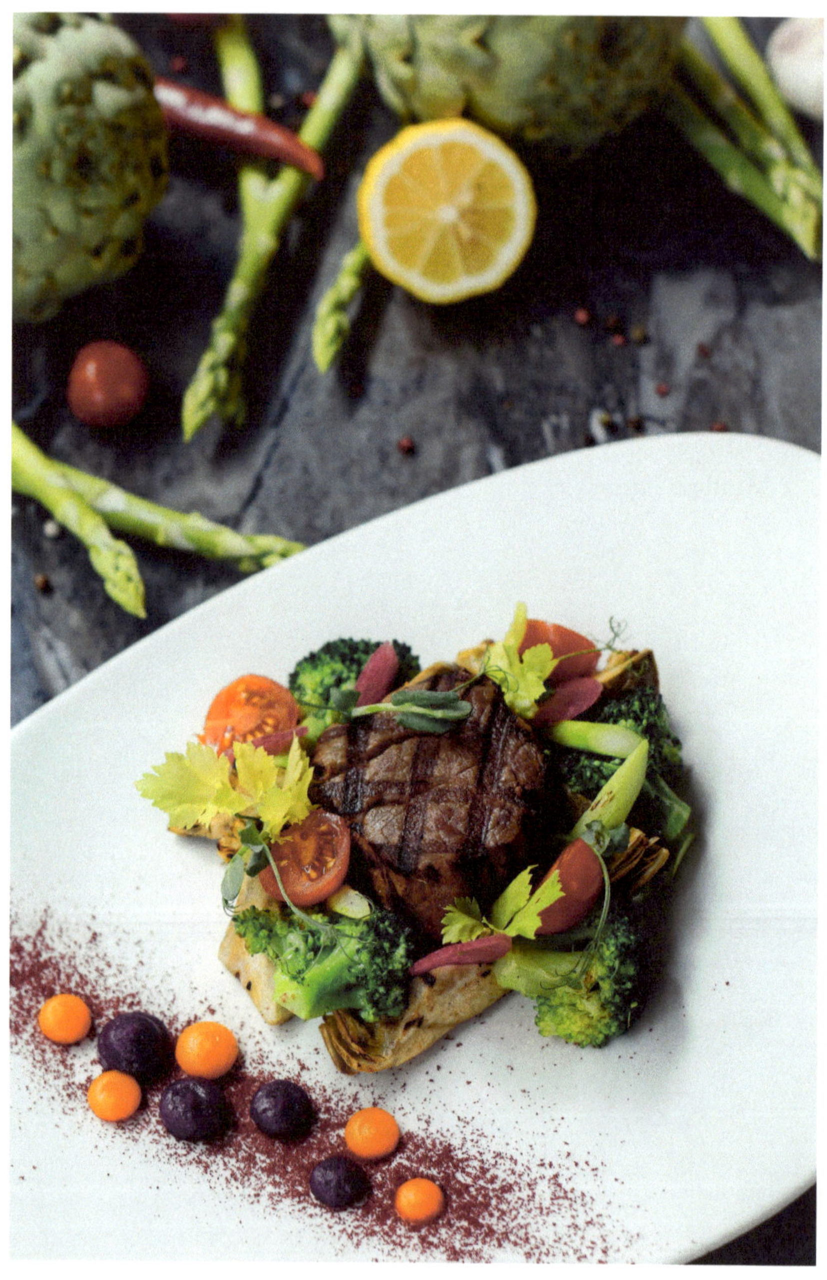

Let's Carry Onward!

Now that you know which foods are carbohydrates, you may feel like, "Well what is left to eat?" I want you to focus on protein, non-starchy vegetables and healthy fats. By the way, FAT IS NOT THE BAD GUY!! I can go on and on about this false, supposedly scientific research, but that may be for another book some other time.

3

Focus on Protein, Healthy Fats and Non-Starchy Vegetables

Protein

Yes, you need protein and it is the major building block of your muscles! If you do not eat enough protein what happens? You lose your muscle that constitutes your overall metabolic health. Muscle burns 10 calories per pound per hour versus burning only 2 calories per pound of fat per hour. You need to prioritize protein intake when you eat, not carbohydrates. Protein builds muscle. Excess carbohydrates build fat. Why would you prioritize what builds fat in your body? I know, it tastes good at the moment. Well so does a savory ribeye! Protein produces a hormone called peptide YY promoting decreased appetite and a feeling of satiety. Protein intake can be approximately 20-25% of your total daily intake. Unless you are a bodybuilder, again, another book for another time.

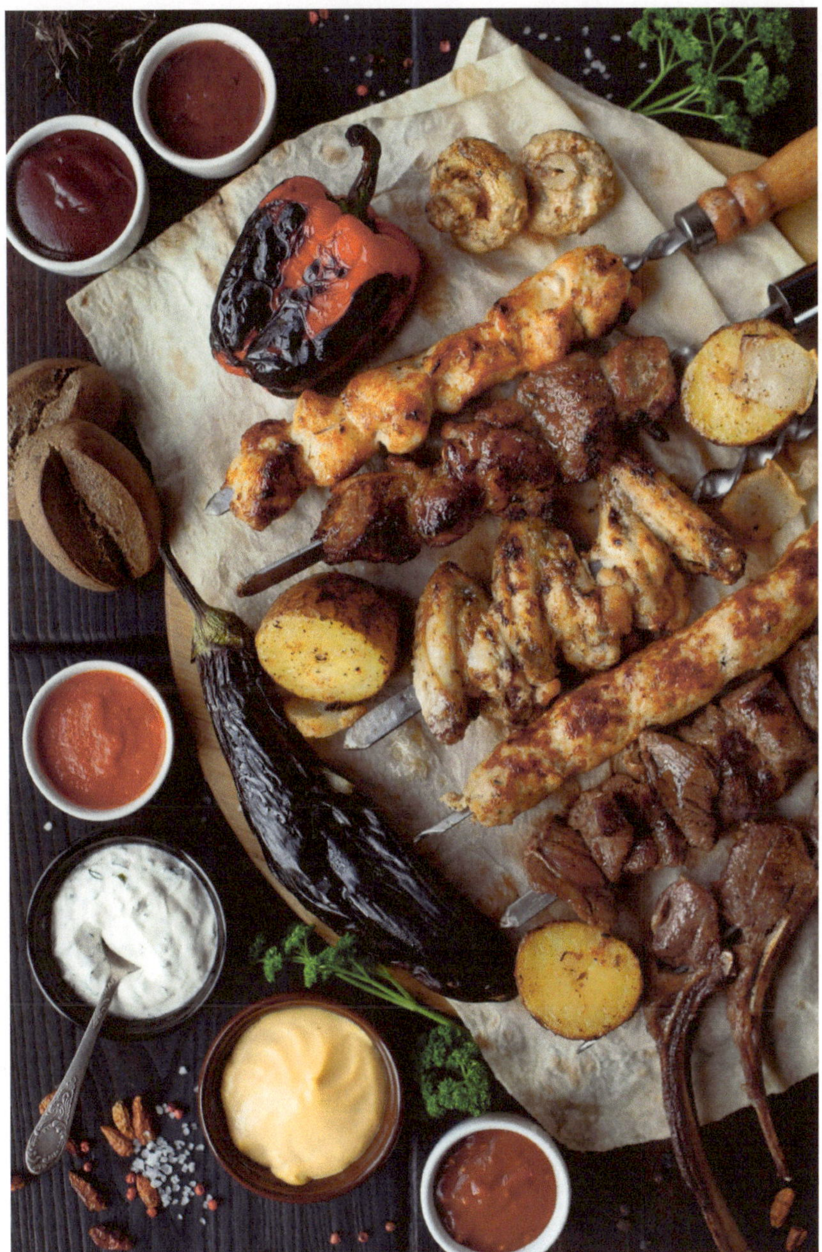

Healthy Fats

Healthy fats such as nuts, seeds, olives, extra-virgin olive oil, salmon and avocado are great sources of healthy fats that are good for your heart and they do not affect your insulin at all! In addition, when you eat fats, they produce a peptide hormone in your body called cholecystokinin contributing to the feeling of satiety in your body. Now you can't go hog wild on fats and consume way over your calorie level. It's okay if fats make up 40% or more of your daily caloric intake. Remember, fats do not affect your insulin levels.

Non-Starchy Vegetables

I love some non-starchy vegetables! In fact, I can eat a whole plate full at one time. These vegetables are rich in vitamins and minerals and contain good fiber with small amounts of carbohydrates. Remember your mom saying, "Eat your vegetables!" I am saying, "Eat your vegetables first!" Whether it's salad or other non-starchy vegetables (broccoli, asparagus, cauliflower, carrots), always try to eat them first at your meal. They provide a fiber barrier for your microbiome and slow down absorption of any carbohydrates you may eat after. Starchy vegetables to limit, containing higher amounts of carbohydrates, include corn, green peas, potatoes and acorn squash. I'm hoping your plate will be filled with mostly protein, salad, other non-starchy vegetables and healthy fats!

4

Low Carb Meal Examples at Restaurants

I spent a lot of time going to restaurants and ordering low carb meals in order to have a helpful teaching source for both my patients and my readers. Both of these pictures are meals I ate at restaurants. The first picture is a fajita meal without the tortillas. The second picture is a burrito bowl over lettuce with no rice. It's amazing how you can eat flavorful meals without hardly any carbohydrates! While still feeling satisfied and full because of eating protein & fats. Yummm! You can refer to my instagram @Carb.Medic.RD for many more low carb restaurant meal examples.

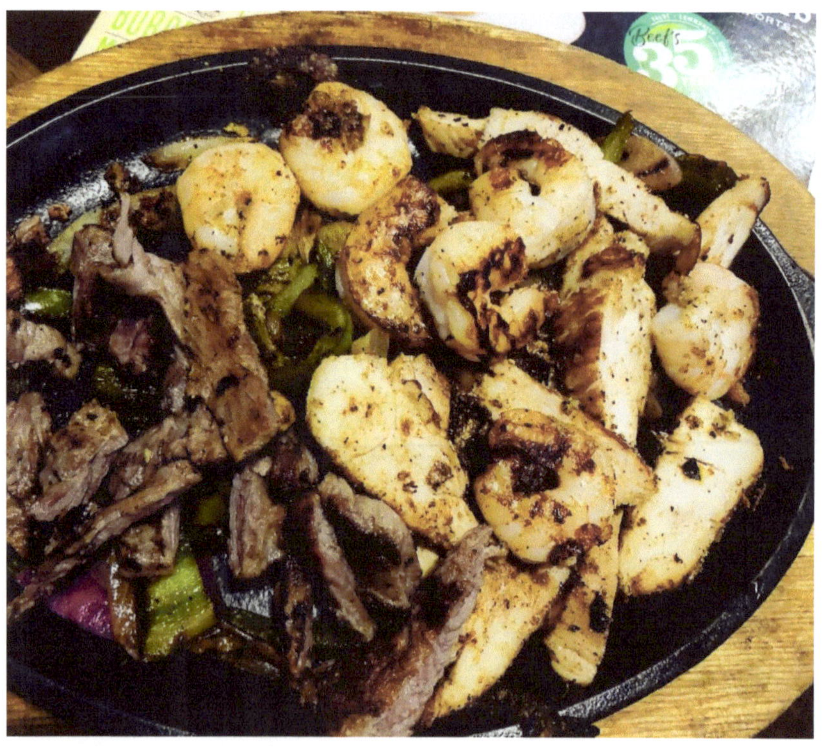

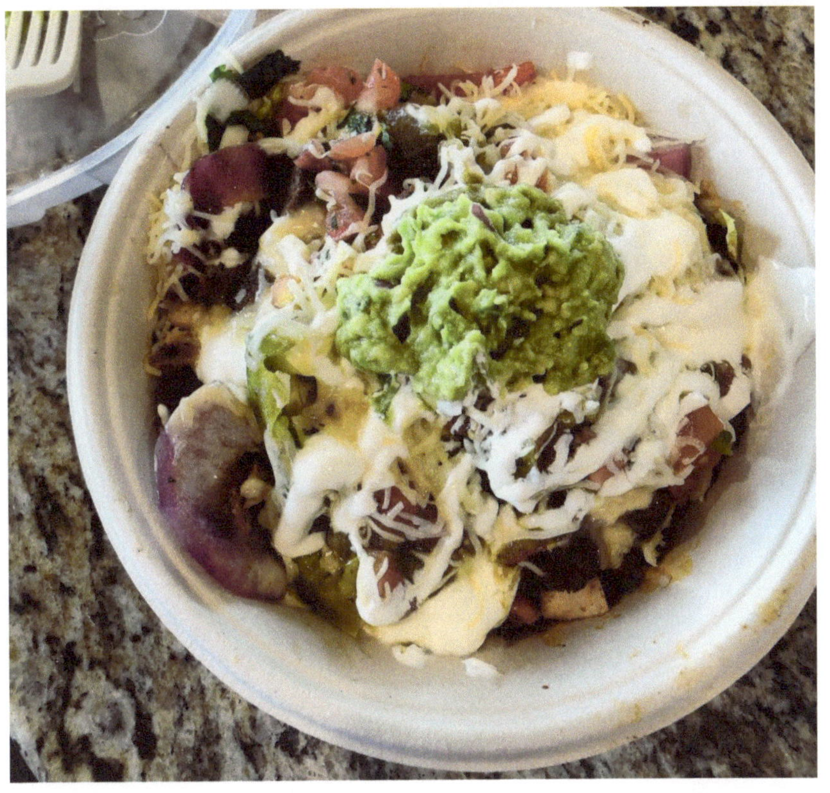

5

Diets Suck

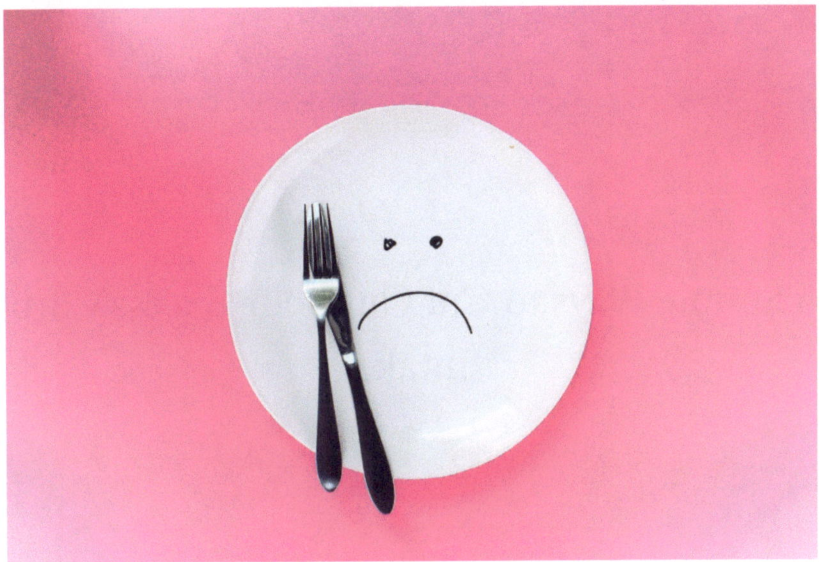

"Die"t

I honestly wish the word diet would just die and erase itself from the planet. We all know every attempt at a diet usually fails. This book will show you 5 easy low carb changes you can make daily that can stick for your lifetime. One of my patients followed the 5 easy steps that changed her life. She came to my office and said, "I can do this everyday and I don't feel like I am on a diet at all!" I cherish those words when I hear my patients say them and my goal is to have everyone that reads my book say those words too! Diets are too stressful and can backfire when it is the only thing on your mind. It can make you more obsessed with food. I am going to show you how you can still eat carbohydrates, prioritizing which ones you are going to eat in a day. There is still a way to eat a variety that tastes so good with low carb intake. Let's get started!

6

5 Simple Ways to Cut Out Your Excess Carb Intake

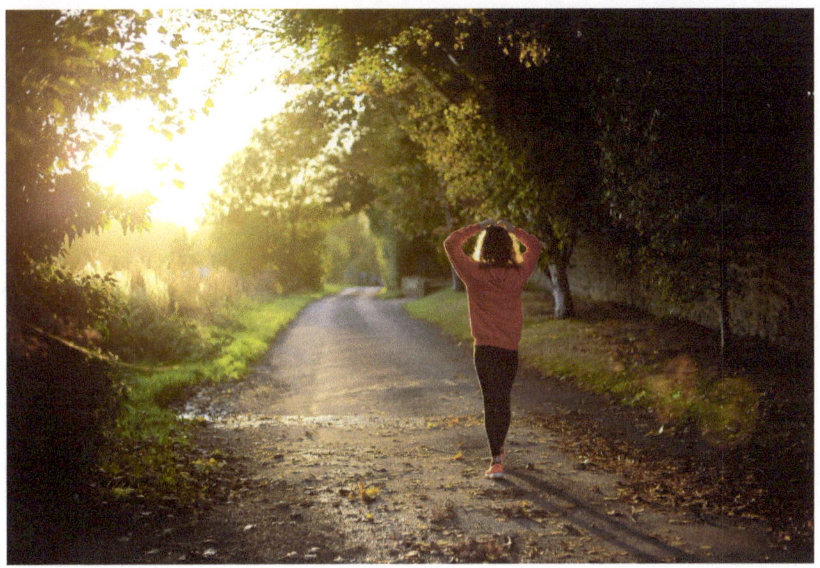

CHANGE #1 Stop Drinking Your Carbohydrates!

- All your drinks should be low carb. Look on your label and if it is over 5 grams of total carbohydrates per serving do not drink it!
- There are approximately 70-80 grams of carbohydrates in 32 ounces of a regular soda. It is easy to drink that much, especially when we get the large size cups at the gas station.
- You may not know that regular lemonade may have 90-100 grams total grams of carbs in 32 ounces. Imagine realizing you have just drank 100% of your total carbs for the day instead of eating them!
- Southern sweet tea! I am from the north, however I have lived in the south for 13 years and there are a lot of sweet tea drinkers down here. A 32 ounce cup of sweet tea can contain up to 140-150 grams total carbs! So not worth it!

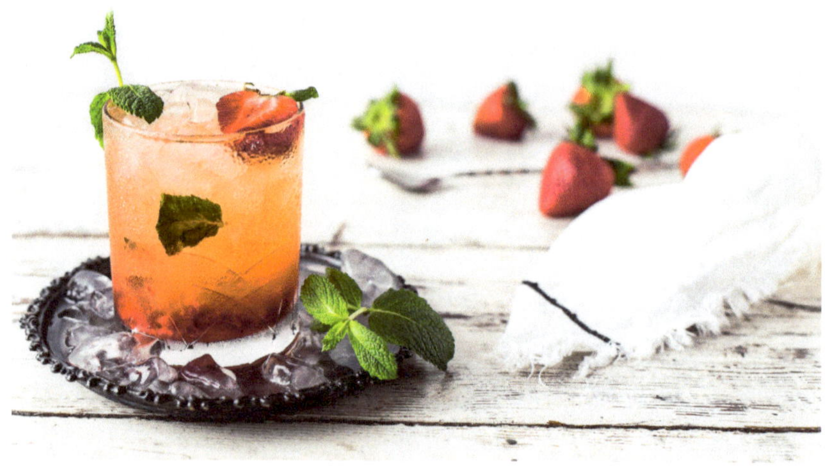

- What about alcohol? Alcohol slows weight loss and your liver prioritizes metabolizing alcohol especially over any food you eat, therefore your food sits in your stomach and is most likely stored later as fat. However, if you choose to indulge, choose low carb beers, non-carb seltzers, skinny margaritas, and liquor with soda water or diet soda. Add sugar substitutes to your drink to make it taste good if need be!

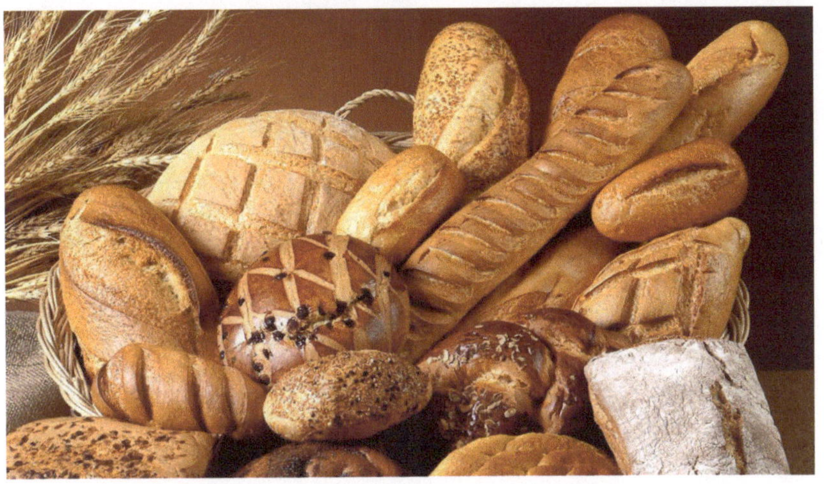

CHANGE #2 Don't Eat Bread at Restaurants!

- Tell your wait staff to keep the bread. They are busy serving tables… they can afford to eat it! Ask the waiter to bring out your side salad right away to take away any hunger pains you may be experiencing. Ask for water and drink a glass to help you not feel as hungry.
- Pretend the wait person sneezed on the bread if it ends up on your table anyway! I tell my patients this trick all the time. If you knew someone sneezed whatever food you really wanted to eat, would you eat it? All my patients say NO WAY!! I'm sure you would too!
- Always order a side salad and eat that first so it keeps you busy and fills you up with good fiber!
- Order protein such as fish, steak, pork or chicken and non-starchy vegetables such as broccoli, carrots, zucchini and asparagus
- Skip the potato, rice, pasta and french fries. If you want carbohydrates, try a sweet potato with only butter. Sweet potato has good fiber and doesn't affect your blood sugars like a russet potato.

CHANGE #3 Toss the Top Bun Please!

- Who invented the hamburger anyway? Where did hamburger buns originate? The hamburger bun, as we know it today, is thought to have been created in the early 20th century. One popular story is that the first hamburger bun was created in 1916 by a fry cook named Walter Anderson, who worked at a diner. At that time processed foods were not readily available like today. Since our society is overwhelmed with processed and high carb foods you have to think twice about eating the whole bun now-a-days.

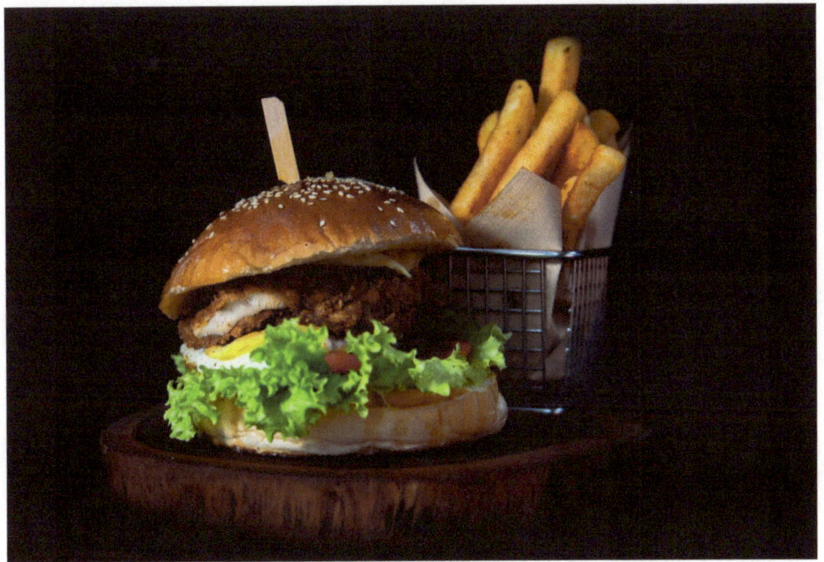

- I'll be honest, my burger without the bun actually tastes better. Have you tried it? The bun takes away from the flavor of the burger.
- Always eat your sandwich, hamburger,etc open-faced and pull as much bread off the bottom as possible. You can order burgers through drive through fast food restaurants without the bun as well as sit down restaurants. It's very common so most of the employees won't look at you weird.
- If you are driving and eating, it's still easy to eat the bunless sandwich when you are on the go! Take the top of the bun off and tear off as much as you can off the bottom. Leave a little left on the bottom to hold the burger or sandwich. Look at all the carbs you just threw out!
- If people look at you strangely, they are jealous and need to read this book haha!

- When you eat fast food, double up on the protein, skip the fries and always at least toss the top bun.
- If you want to save a dollar on the "combo" meal, what's important is saving your body from carb overload. Order a carb free drink; diet soda, diet lemonade or unsweetened tea. If you order a salad, the dressing should be low carb like ranch. If you order a chicken sandwich or burger, toss the top bun and eat it open faced. If you get french fries, eat one or two and pretend your child sneezed on the rest.
- Do you ever feel like your chicken wrap is too much tortilla and not enough chicken, cheese and vegetables?
- If you order a wrap, open it and rip away all the extra that you don't need to save on carbs. The tortilla is usually "extra wrapped." Tear off the extra to save on your carb intake. If you order fajitas at a restaurant, eat the chicken, steak and sauteed vegetables and limit your tortilla to one or none.
- You can do this with enchiladas as well. If you are making enchiladas at home, tear off the extra tortilla before you bake them. You can also use zero carb tortillas instead.

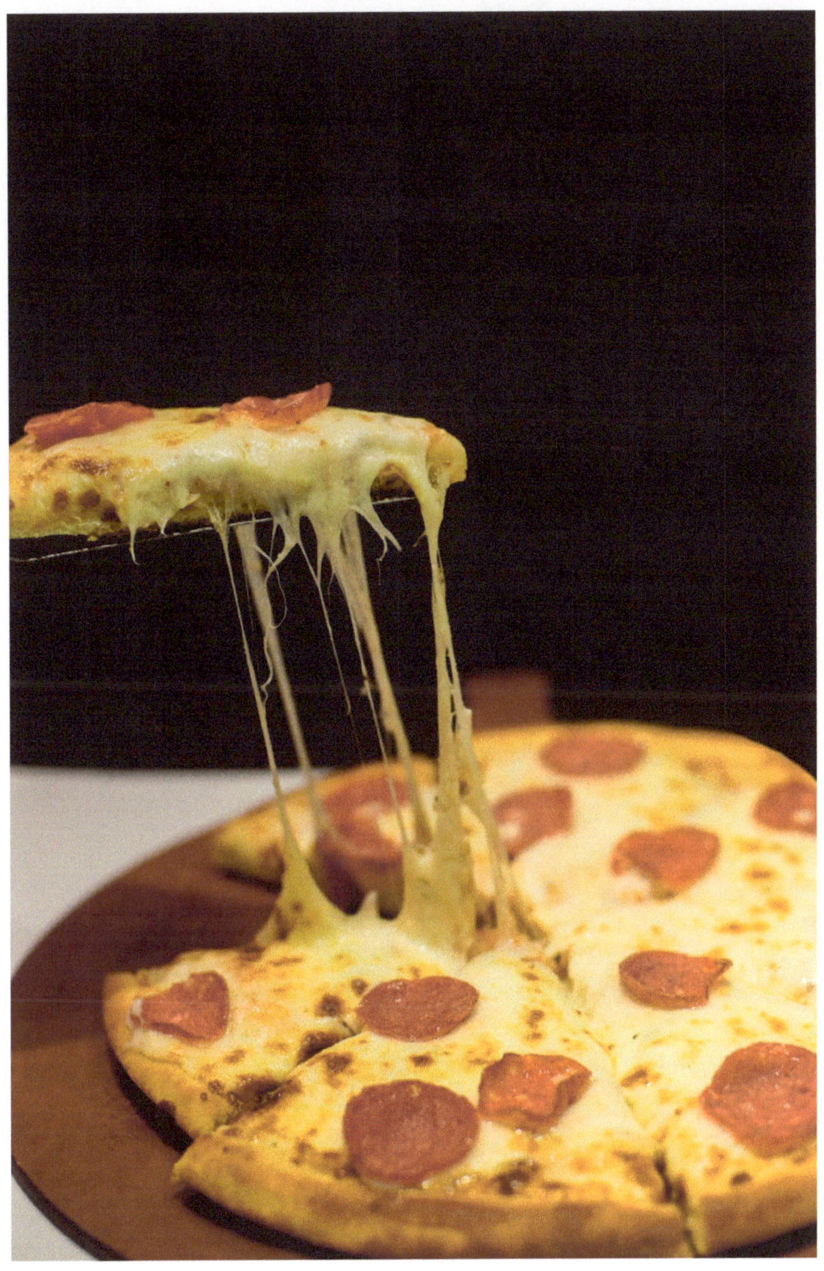

CHANGE #4 Pizza Crust Matters!

- Thin crust has the least amount of carbs compared to pan or Old Chicago style. If you are eating a thicker crust, try eating one slice with a side salad. If you don't have a salad, eat one slice and the toppings off the second slice.
- Some restaurants may offer a cauliflower crust. I go to a pizza restaurant where I order the cauliflower crust for my pizza. The restaurant makes cheese breadsticks for me with the cauliflower crust. I also had them read the label on the cauliflower crust box to make sure indeed it is low carb. Before I knew it my patients were going to the same restaurant ordering the same thing and the low carb cauliflower crust became a hit. The best thing is that it tastes delicious too!

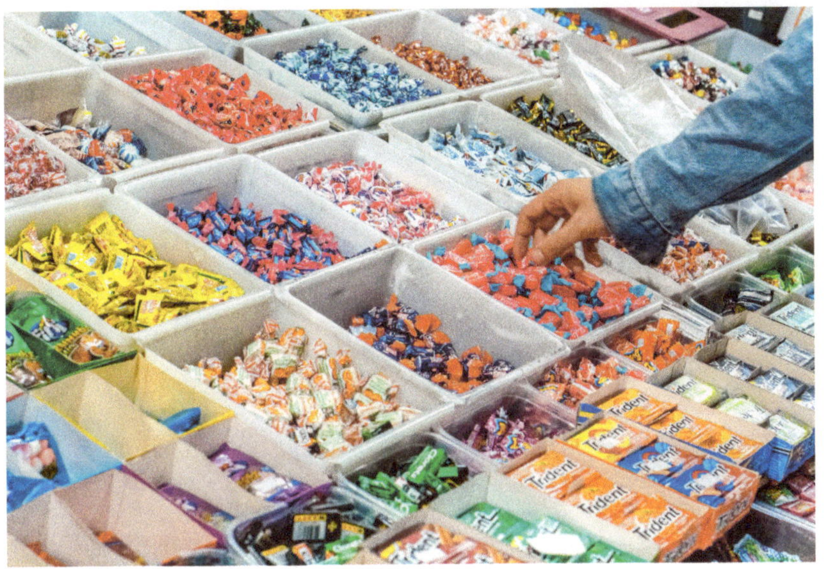

CHANGE #5 Keep Your Junk Food Out of Reach!

- The more accessible your favorite junk foods are to you at home, the more you will eat them. Are you going to go in your car late at night to go get what you are craving? Or will you find something that will curb your craving that you won't binge on?
- Keep "treat" foods in your home that are keto friendly. There are plenty of these products in the stores.
- If you want fruit, make sure it is berries such as strawberries, blackberries, raspberries or blueberries.
- Stay clear of cereals in your home. Most are full of sugar and carbs and people tend to eat the whole box in one sitting. I call cereal a

"trigger" food for many of my patients. Once you start it's hard to stop eating it. It was one of my trigger foods in college. I haven't had cereal in my house for years. Not even for my kids.

- Keep regular bread out of the house. Choose low carb breads and tortillas.
- A healthy handful of nuts and seeds are a good option of healthy fat, protein and fiber.
- Planning ahead for your week of eating helps. Grill a bunch of protein ahead of time so you have it for the week.
- Pick up some of those microwaveable non-starchy vegetables bags from the frozen isle in the grocery store
- Tadah! You have quick, low carb easy meals for the week.

7

Conclusion

Let's Be Real!

I know that not eating any junk food ever…is not reality. What I am asking you is if you have a craving for ice cream or want to eat a piece of cake, prepare your daily carb intake for that. Keep your carb intake low for the rest of the day by eating mostly protein and non-starchy vegetables. I want this to be a way of life for you. I tell my patients it's prioritizing your carb intake for the day. I love to eat sweets & chips too! I prioritize my carbs just like I am teaching you. I don't feel deprived at all…I want you to feel the same!

Wrapping it Up!

In conclusion, I hope this book gives you simple guidance on how to choose low carb foods and not feel like it is stressful or depriving you in any way. I have learned through my own research that cutting back on your daily carb intake significantly has a positive affect on your metabolic health. It is scientifically known that excess carbohydrate intake can increase your risk for many diseases such as diabetes, heart disease, Alzheimer's and obesity. The good news is you may reverse some of these diseases with decreased carbohydrate intake.

Your goal is to keep your insulin levels as low as possible throughout the day. I am an advocate of fasting during the day, keeping insulin levels low. If you are interested in fasting I would recommend Doctor Jason Fung's books on it. Remember that your blood only needs one teaspoon of glucose daily. Your liver and muscles store glucose up to a certain

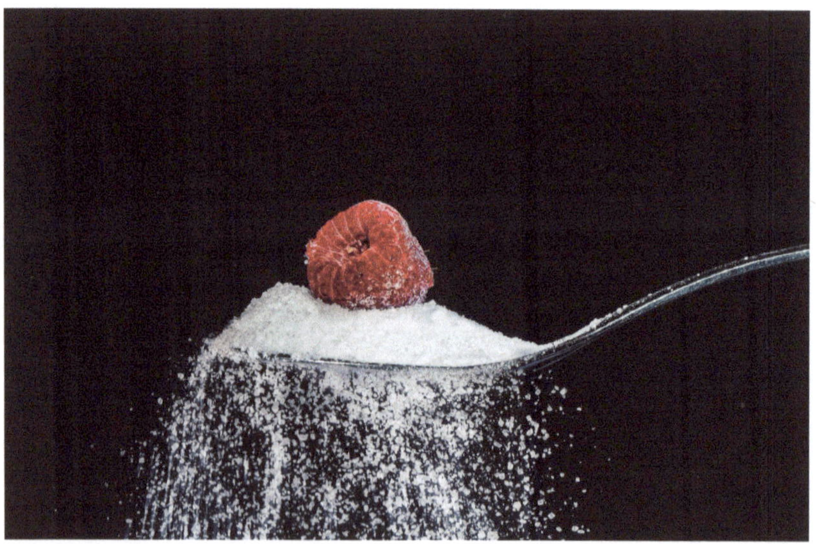

amount. What happens to all that extra glucose floating around in your blood? It is parked as fat storage. Keep your carb intake low. Your body doesn't need to process all those extra carbohydrates. Be good to your body! I suggest not going beyond 25-30% of your total calories as carbohydrates. Everyone has different individual low carb daily recommendations. In general, women should stay under 100 grams and men under 200 grams of total carbohydrates per day.

Again, if you would like to learn more about how to choose low carb meals while eating out, whether fast food or dining out, go to my instagram page @Carb.Medic.RD. I have example pictures of low carb meals from various restaurants. I also share how many grams of carbohydrates are in each meal.

As far as exercise, if you start living a low carb life, I recommend adding in exercise that doesn't stress you out and that you can tolerate and enjoy. You won't want to exercise if you dread doing it every day. Strength training is highly recommended as tolerated. Remember that building your muscles will change your body composition and you will be more metabolically healthy. Cardio exercise is good for your heart, decreases stress levels and does use up some of your reserved glucose. Most importantly it is important for your mental health. It makes you feel good! I recommend doing a combination of cardio and strength training. Don't over do your exercise because if you put too much stress on your body, your cortisol hormone will increase. Cortisol will store fat on you too!

One more thing is to get good sleep! If you don't sleep well, your cortisol levels will increase. When you are tired you tend to eat more thinking it will make you have more energy and keep you awake. This can be further from the truth, especially if you are trying to stay awake with carbohydrates. This will spike your blood sugars and then you will feel terrible and think you need to eat more. It's a vicious cycle!

Today, I am so glad I am not living in that vicious cycle of binging on carbs and binging on exercise. I was chasing my carbs and was out-of-control. I felt terrible and it took me years to break the cycle. When I look back I would consider myself, at that time, to be an exercise bulimic. Today I fast most of the day but make sure that I include enough protein and non-starchy vegetables. I do eat carbs, sometimes the junk kind, but it's not anything like it used to be! Now I do strength training most days but it's only 10-15 minutes a day. I will also go out on very short runs, maybe 1-2 miles. Let it be known it's actually a "run/walk" not just a run. I was a runner all my life and never thought I would be a "run/walker" but here I am!

Lastly, my hope for you is that you will find some peace in your lifestyle by reading my book. Make sure whatever changes you choose, that they are not stressful or impossible. That is not reality. You deserve to have health and live a long prosperous life. We all struggle and I highly respect those of you that seek out extra support as you need. You deserve to be happy and healthy. I believe God's greatest gift he gave me is to be your biggest cheerleader! YOU GOT THIS!

I would LOVE & APPRECIATE it if you would leave a favorable review of my quick read book on Amazon and how it has positively impacted your life! I will be writing more books in the near future and would love for you to read those as well!

Thank you for reading my book!

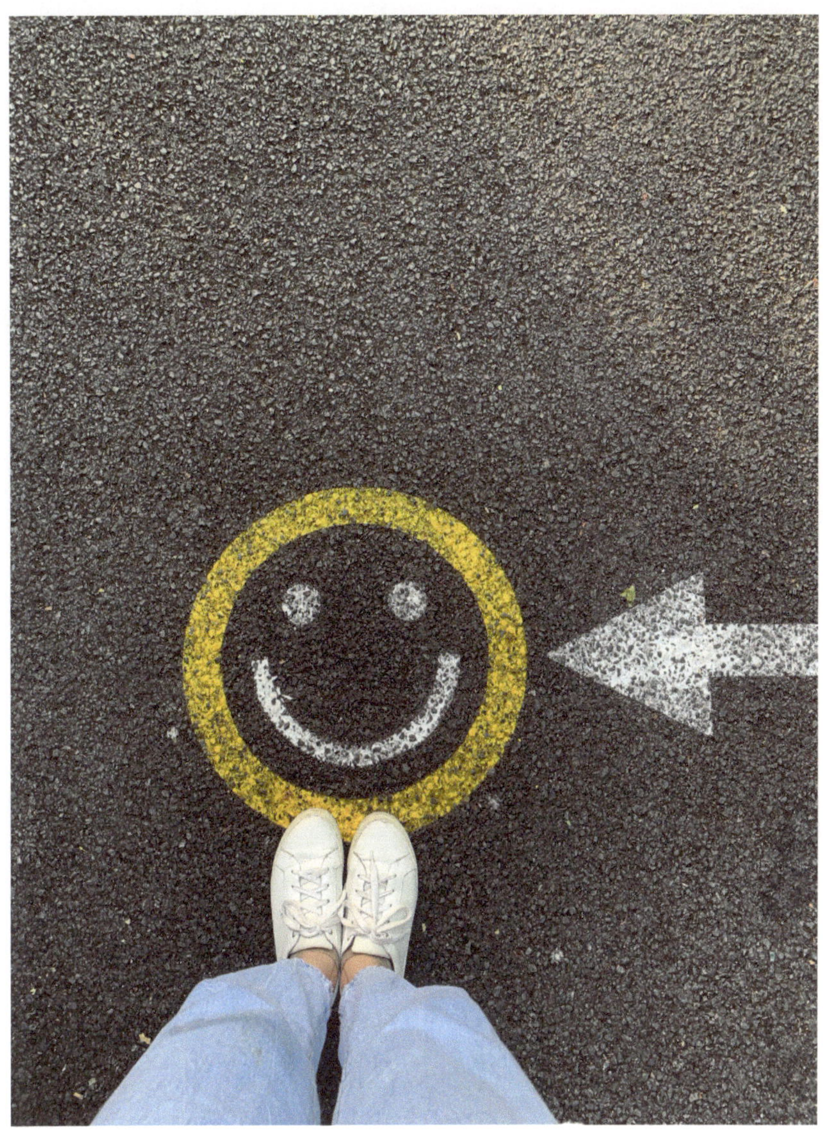

RESOURCES

Professional, C. C. M. (n.d.). *Cholecystokinin.* Cleveland Clinic. https://my.clevelandclinic.org/health/body/23110-cholecystokinin

Wikipedia contributors. (2024, June 9). *History of the hamburger in the United States.* Wikipedia. https://en.wikipedia.org/wiki/History_of_the_hamburger_in_the_United_States

Karra, E., Chandarana, K., & Batterham, R. L. (2009). The role of peptide YY in appetite regulation and obesity. *Journal of Physiology, 587*(1), 19–25. https://doi.org/10.1113/jphysiol.2008.164269

The Obesity Code — Dr. Jason Fung. (n.d.). Dr. Jason Fung. https://www.doctorjasonfung.com/the-obesity-code